Fight Cancer With Juicing

Use the Power of Natural Juice

to

Help Prevent and Fight Off Cancer

RON KNESS

Contents

Disclaimer

This publication is for informational purposes only and is not intended as medical advice. Medical advice should always be obtained from a qualified medical professional for any health conditions or symptoms associated with them.

Every possible effort has been made in preparing and researching this material. We make no warranties with respect to the accuracy, applicability of its contents or any omissions.

Juicing for Health

Juicing is a healthy practice that has allowed millions of people to boost their nutrition. Juicing fruits and vegetables provides you important antioxidants, which scavenge for oxygen free radicals that can damage cellular structures, including DNA. When DNA is damaged, it can result in mutations that lead to cancer.

Well-balanced nutrition from a variety of healthy whole foods helps support and maintain on-going good health, and experts agree that nutrition plays a key role in preventing chronic and terminal illness.

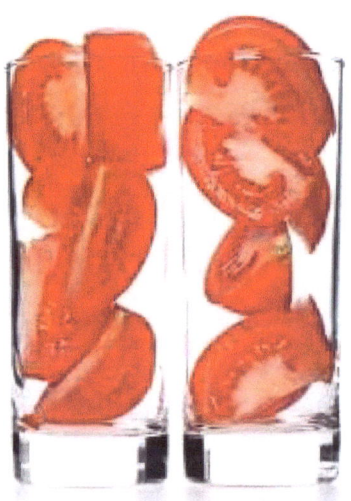

Juicing is practiced by millions around the world and it is an easy and convenient way to get plant nutrition into the body to do its magic.

When juicing is done right, that is when the majority of your juice blends is comprised of vegetables and very low sugar fruit, you can easily boost your nutritional intake thereby improving your health and lower your risks for cancer.

Best Juicing Vegetables

There are several raw vegetables that are especially recommended for reducing risks for various types of cancer. Many people also utilize these vegetables as a support in fighting cancer once a diagnosis has been made.

Of course, no scientific evidence exists that juicing or eating these

vegetables can cure cancer, or guarantee that you will never get it, but it is true that healthy nutrient rich juices can boost immunity, promote energy, which is often drained during cancer treatments and boost your overall health.

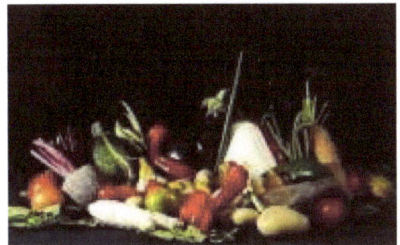

Furthermore, scientific research has found promising results in certain vegetables playing a key role in cancer prevention.

Cruciferous Vegetables

Cruciferous vegetables are part of the Brassica genus plant family. These vegetables are rich in key nutrients, including carotenoids, such as lutein, beta-carotene, and zeaxanthin. They are also rich sources of key vitamins, including vitamins C, E, and K along with folate and minerals.

Moreover, these gems of nature provide a group of substances known as glucosinolates, which are chemicals that contain sulfur. It is the sulfur that gives some of these vegetables their bitter flavor, like that in greens.

According to the National Cancer Institute, animal studies and lab grown cell experiments have identified numerous potential ways in which glucosinolates can help in preventing cancer:

- Protect cells from DNA damage
- Ability to inactivate carcinogens
- Hold antiviral, anti-inflammatory and antibacterial properties
- Induce apoptosis or cell death
- Hinder tumor blood vessel formation and migration, which is required for metastasis

The following section details some of the cruciferous vegetables that are best for juicing.

Broccoli

Broccoli contains high levels of sulforaphane, a very potent compound that increases the body's protective enzymes and flushes out cancer-causing chemicals. Juice the whole vegetable, including the stems, leaves, and florets as they hold key nutrients.

Cabbage

Another member of the cruciferous family of vegetables that provides powerful antioxidants including, vitamins A and C and the phytonutrients, zeaxanthin, isothiocyanates, thiocyanates, lutein, and sulforaphane that stimulate detoxifying enzymes, fight oxidative stress and may offer protection from prostate, colon, and even breast cancers.

In addition, sulforaphane selectively targets cancer stem cells that may prevent cancer from spreading or even recurring.

Cabbage juice is probably not the tastiest on its own, but can be added to delicious cancer fighting blends that include, kale, green apples, berries, and beets.

Kale

According to the National Cancer Institute, kale is yet another valuable cruciferous vegetable that has promise in helping humans fight the battle against cancer.

Kale is rich in important nutrients, such as lutein, zeaxanthin, vitamins C, E, and K; folate; and minerals. Kale also contains glucosinolates, or sulfur-containing chemicals. While the folate found in kale does not have a direct impact on cancer treatment, it does help to reduce the risk of complications from cancer and its treatment by lowering risks for heart disease.

Kale and beets are rich sources of potassium, which is an electrolyte that helps regulate fluid in the body, move nutrients into the cells, and remove waste from cells, and supports the communication between nerves and muscles.

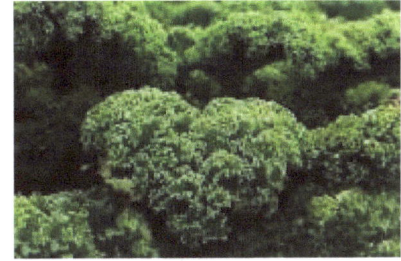

While potassium does not have a direct effect on preventing cancer, it may be beneficial depending upon medications that are prescribed during cancer treatment and side effects that result from treatment, ask your doctor.

While human studies have shown mixed results, it is 100% safe to say that kale is a nutrient rich plant food that is 100% recommended as part of a daily balanced diet and should the cancer fighting promise materialize that is just icing on the cake.

Kale juices great, and blends wonderfully with many different nutritious fruits and vegetables.

It may be an acquired taste for some, but adding lemon or lime juice, and a green apple to kale makes it very tasty.

Other Cruciferous Vegetables:

- Arugula
- Bok Choy
- Brussels Sprouts
- Collard Greens
- Radishes
- Rutabaga
- Turnips
- Watercress

Carrots

Carrots contain natural compounds, poly-acetylenes that are only found in carrots, but also ginseng and that protect the plant from pests and disease.

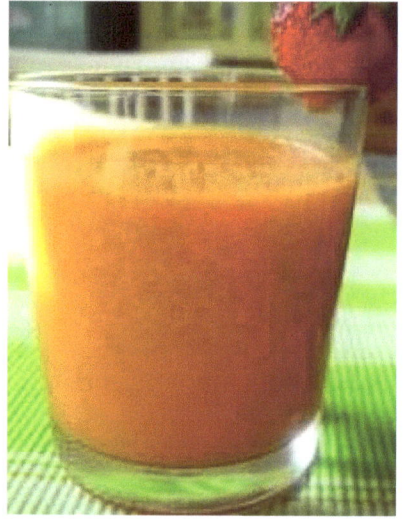

Various tests have shown poly-acetylenes to fight inflammation and cancer, and has shown to reduce cancer growth in rats. Carrots also contain beta-carotene, alpha carotene, vitamin E, and other cancer fighting nutrients.

Carrots are higher in sugar than green vegetables, so watch your juicing intake. Carrot juice blends great with kale, cabbage, and green apples.

Beets

These colorful purple gems of nature contain betacyanin that researchers believe could protect against the development of cancer cells, and may possibly reduce risks for inflammation, which promotes malignancy.

Beets are wonderful for juicing and **a great blend is 3 small beets, 1 cucumber, 1 handful of spinach and an orange**.

Turmeric

Turmeric is not technically a vegetable, but a spice that is often used in Asian and Indian cooking and belongs to the ginger family. It is grown in Asian countries and has been used for centuries in herbal medicine.

Turmeric contains curcumin that is believed by experts to have exceptional anti-inflammatory abilities, which makes it effective for fighting cancer because most diseases are caused by and thrive under a state of chronic and long-term inflammation, according to a biochemist at The University of Texas M. D. Anderson Cancer Center, Bharat B. Aggarwal, PhD. Recent studies found curcumin to interfere with cell-signaling pathways that suppress the transformation, proliferation, and invasion of cancer cells.

According to Cancer Research UK, curcumin was found to stop pre-cancerous changes to becoming cancer when given to 25 patients with pre-cancerous changes in different organs in a phase 1 clinical trial.

Analytical research has found that certain type of cancer rates are lowest in countries where curcumin is consumed at levels of about 100 to 200 mg a day regularly.

Numerous lab studies on cancer cells have found curcumin to have anticancer effects, as it not only killed cancer cells but also prevented their growth. These studies found these effects to be most profound on skin, bowel, breast, and stomach cancer cells.

A 2007 study done in the United States, found that a combination of curcumin and chemotherapy killed more bowel cancer cells than chemotherapy alone. Another 2007 US study of mice found that curcumin helped to stop the spread of breast cancer cells to other parts of the body.

How To Use In Juicing

Fresh turmeric can be juiced along with other fruits and vegetables. Another option is to add 1 or 2 teaspoons of the ground spice into your juices and enjoy the health boost!

Garlic

The phytochemicals found in garlic help to stop the formation of nitrosamines, which are carcinogens formed in the stomach, and under certain conditions in the intestines.

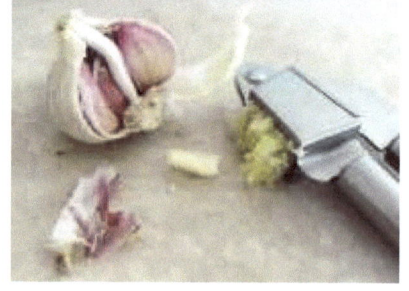

Garlic is a vegetable that's part of the Allium class of bulb-shaped plants that also features leeks, onions, chives, and scallions.

Garlic contains an unusually high amount of sulfur along with flavonoids, arginine, oligosaccharides, and selenium.

Garlic's pungent odor and flavor stems from the sulfur compounds, which are formed from allicin, a major precursor of the bioactive compounds in garlic formed when garlic cloves are crushed or chopped.

These bioactive compounds are defined as elements in food other than those needed for basic nutrition, but are responsible for changes in health.

According to the National Cancer Institute, several multidisciplinary studies of population groups that investigate causes, spread of, incidence and effect of certain health-related interventions, nutritional intakes, or environmental exposures, have shown a relationship between increases in intake of garlic and a reduction in risks for cancers of the pancreas, breast, stomach, colorectal, esophagus and colon.

The Iowa Women's Study has looked into whether diet, body fat distribution along with other risk factors contribute to cancer rates in older women. The study has found that women who eat the highest amounts of garlic reduced their risk for colon cancer by 50% cancer as compared to women whose consumption levels were much lower.

Higher intakes of onion and garlic were associated with a reduced risk of intestinal cancer in the European Prospective Investigation into Cancer and Nutrition, which involves men and women from 10 different countries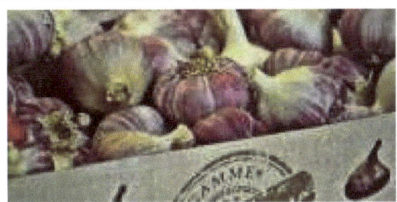

Numerous population studies conducted in China that centered on intake of garlic and cancer risk have found a strong connection between garlic and lower cancer rates.

One of these studies, found that regular and frequent intake of garlic reduced risk for esophageal and stomach cancers and risk factors grew with higher consumption levels

Another one of the studies in China found that high intake of garlic and onions reduced risk for stomach cancer.

Yet another study found that the greater the intake of garlic and scallions, meaning more than 10 grams daily versus less than 2.2 grams per day was associated with about a 50% reduction in prostate cancer risk.

A study in France found that higher intake of garlic was linked with a statistically significant reduction in risk for breast cancer.

A study conducted in the San Francisco Bay discovered a 54% lower risk for pancreatic cancer in people who had a high intake of garlic versus those who ate much less.

How To Use In Juicing

Juiced garlic is very potent, but just a little bit is all you need, with 1 to 2 cloves added to any of the other vegetables mentioned, and even fruits, like green apples or tomatoes. The other ingredients will mask the pungent flavor allowing you to get your pure raw garlic nutrition without sacrificing taste.

A nice savory juice includes, garlic, tomatoes, cabbage, celery or zucchini, shallots or any onion and red peppers, makes for a great meatless lunch or dinner.

Of course, if you can stand it, go ahead and a get a shot of straight garlic juice daily! Besides cancer, it will help you fight the cold, flu, allergies, sinusitis along with various other respiratory disorders, and it has significant cardiovascular benefits due to its natural ability to reduce vascular inflammation and blood clotting.

Ginger

According to WebMd, researchers have found ginger able to kill cancer cells in two ways.

- In a process called apoptosis, cancer cells kill themselves without harming surrounding healthy cells.

- In another process known as autophagy, cancer cells are duped into digesting themselves as described by J. Rebecca Liu, an assistant professor of obstetrics and gynecology at the University of Michigan doing extensive research on ginger's effects on ovarian cancer cells.

While only preliminary, and animal and human trials are still needed, the research is promising because patient's with ovarian cancer develop resistance to chemotherapy drugs, so ginger's ability to kill cancer cells in more than one way may prove useful.

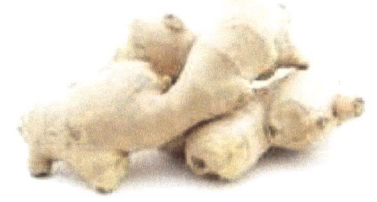

The Comprehensive Cancer Center at the University of Michigan Health system does not recommend ginger supplements, but does recommend fresh ginger in dietary form not only for its potential cancer fighting role, but also because it is healthy in other ways and works great for nausea.

How To Use In Juicing

Ginger adds a fresh, floral, and crisp flavor to a variety of juice blends, or if you really love it, you can take a small shot of it on its own.

Peel a small piece of fresh ginger with a spoon and add to your juicer, typically a 1" inch piece is more than enough. While ginger does not produce a lot of juice, it does add a lot of flavor so a little goes a long way.

Caution: Avoid excessive amounts if you take blood-thinners or diabetes medication, ask your doctor.

Best Juicing Fruits

Fruit juices can also prevent cancer or even help fight cancer once a diagnosis is made. The American Institute For Cancer Research recommends the following raw fruits to aid in the fight against cancer.

Purple Grapes

Both grapes and juice of grapes including the skin are excellent

sources of resveratrol, which is a phytochemical from a group of phytochemicals known as polyphenols.

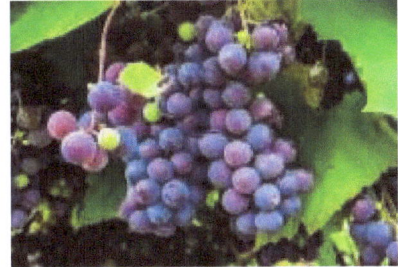

Numerous studies have suggested that polyphenols and especially resveratrol is a powerful antioxidant that in lab studies has prevented particular damage known to trigger the cancer process in tissues, cells, and animal models.

How To Use In Juicing

Make sure to juice the whole grape, as the skin holds much of the resveratrol. Blend with vegetables for a powerful healthy juice.

Blueberries

These blue beauties contain cancer fighting phytochemicals, ellagic acid, and anthocyanins. The Institute reports that cell studies of these compounds showed these nutrients to decrease the growth of cancer cells and also to stimulate self-destruction of breast, prostate, mouth, and, colon cancer cells.

Centrifugal juicers cannot juice berries and grapes, but masticating and singer-auger juicers can.

How To Use In Juicing

To use blueberries it is best to blend them, then strain over a bowl with a spout (for easier pouring) to remove the pulp, or better yet leave the pulp and pour the juice and pulp into your main juice, like a blend of kale and other greens. This results in a type of smoothie juice blend.

Watermelon

Watermelon has loads of lycopene, one of the more potent antioxidant shown in research to protect against prostate cancer.

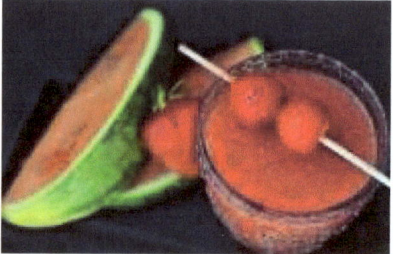

Watermelon is also one of the best fruits for weight control as it really satisfies the sweet tooth with just 49 calories per 2 cup serving.

Since it is one of the lower sugar fruits, it is ideal for juicing and juices quite well.

How To Use In Juicing

Juicing watermelon depends on your juicer model; check the manual to see how much prep is required, for example if the skin should be removed.

Peaches

The peach gets is bright orange color from beta-carotene that helps to reduce inflammation, protect DNA, boost immunity function and plays a key role in controlling cell growth in a way that reduces risks for cancer.

Strawberries

Strawberries contain ellagic acid, a key phytochemical in decreasing growth of cancer cells and stimulating soft-destruction of cancer cells, such as those in the breast, colon, prostate and mouth.

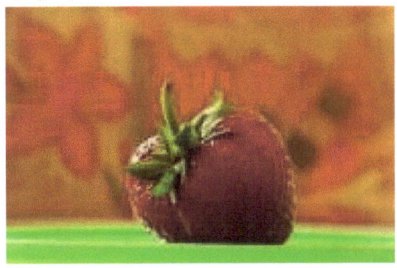

Furthermore, studies have shown that ellagic acid uses several different cancer-fighting methods simultaneously, as it acts as an antioxidant, slows reproduction of cancer cells, and supports the body in deactivating specific carcinogens.

How To Use In Juicing

Strawberries are more difficult to juice, depending on the model of your juicer. If you have a smoothie maker you can use that or mash them up and add them in after your main juice is ready; this also allows you to get more fiber intake from these healthy berries. A food processor or blender works great too. Strawberries go great with a kale, broccoli, and spinach or any greens.

Apples

Apples contain potent phytochemicals that protect cells from cancer-inducing oxidative damage.

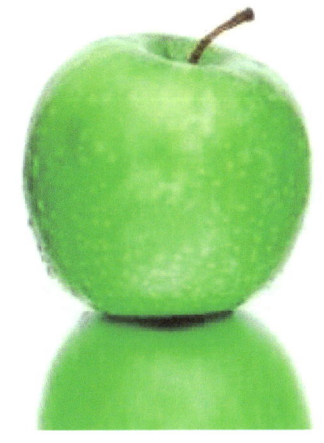

According to the American Institute For Cancer Research, apples can help prevent the start of cancer growth, stop continued tumor growth, and promote cancer cell death.

Laboratory studies conducted by Dr. Rui Hai Liu showed the phytochemicals in apples to suppress breast cancer tumor growth.

The Institute recommends eating one or more apples per day as it is associated with lower risks for both colon and lung cancer in numerous large-scale human studies that evaluated apple consumption and cancer incidence.

How To Use In Juicing

Apples juice great and are a fantastic complimentary flavor to many vegetables. Check your juicer's manual on necessary prep required as they do vary, for example, some allow you to add a whole apple down the feed chute, while others require cutting.

Choose green apples, as they are lowest in sugar.

Tomatoes

One of the best dietary sources of lycopene, a carotenoid that plays a key role in cancer prevention and was found to stop endometrial cancer (causes almost 8,000 deaths each year) cell growth in a study in Nutrition and Cancer.

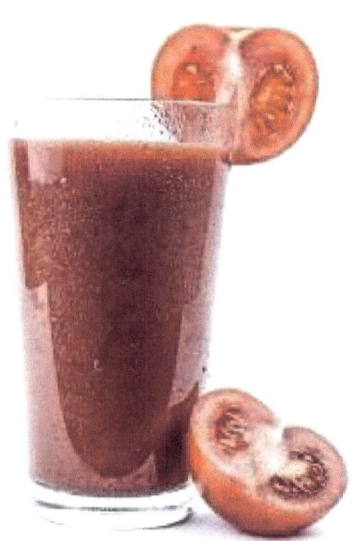

How To Use In Juicing

Juice your own tomatoes for a refreshing, healthy and tangy juice treat! Add garlic to tomato juice, it is a fantastic combination.

Flavor Enhancers for Juice

Some juices are bland on their own, but can be spiced up with the addition of some flavor. Here is a list of some of the more popular things people use for a zestier flavor:

- ✓ Lemons and limes are great additions to your juice blends as they add fresh and tangy flavor and enhance the flavor of green vegetables, especially for those who do not find them palatable.
- ✓ Hot peppers can be juiced if you like spicy flavor.
- ✓ Fresh mint is a wonderful flavor for most any juice blend.
- ✓ You can stir in any spice you like once your juice is ready.
- ✓ Many herbs, like basil, and oregano can be juiced to get flavor and their respective health benefits.
- ✓ Add ice to make a more cool and refreshing drink.
- ✓ Some juicers allow you to make frozen drinks, a great idea for summer.
- ✓ Look up recipes online or in books to add variety to your juicing habit.
- ✓ Experiment with different fruits and vegetables to find you favorite blends. This is key is sticking with this healthy new habit!

Watch The Sugar Intake

Approximately 88% or more of all your juice blends should be vegetables, and 20% or less fruit.

Generally, best juicing practices prescribe the use of more vegetables than fruits as fruit is high in sugar. Even though it is natural sugar, it is still sugar.

Since it takes much more of the fruit to juice as it would if you were eating fruit whole, those who get into the habit of juicing more fruit than vegetables can easily triple or quadruple the recommended daily sugar intake for adults, not to mention calories with just one glass of juice.

Juicing When You Already Have Cancer

As part of your cancer fighting juicing diet, you should not eat any poultry, fish, meat, or dairy products. Cooked foods such as these prevent the immune system from maximally fighting off cancer cells. Instead, the immune system must spend its time dealing with the effects of cooked foods, pesticides, chemical supplements, fungicides, herbicides, toxins, and the hormones found in meat and dairy products. This prevents the immune system from fighting off cancer cells. Of course, you should consult with your doctor before making any dietary changes.

Don't eat a lot of fruits or vegetables that contain a lot of sugar unless they are one of the cancer fighting fruits and vegetables listed above. Carrot juice, for example, has a lot of sugar in it that is easily taken up by cancer cells. Along with the sugar, the cancer cells take up the cancer fighting nutrients from the carrots and are killed by the nutrients.

Juicing can be beneficial as a way to combat cancer when you already have the disease. When you are being treated for cancer, things like digestive issues, chewing, and swallowing are already problems you may be dealing with.

By juicing fruits and vegetables, you do not have to chew your food and the food is easily digested. You shouldn't go on an exclusively juiced diet, however, because it can result in weight loss, which is already a problem in people who have cancer.

Besides juicing, you should be eating at least five servings of whole colorful fruits and vegetables daily. You can eat these fruits and vegetables whole or juice some of them if you are having problems with digestion or swallowing.

Ideally, though, you should be eating the first five servings of fruits and vegetables, only juicing those you eat beyond that.

Tips on Juicing in Support of Cancer Treatment

Here are a few tips to juicing when you have cancer.

- **Eat more vegetables than fruits.** Vegetables contain the most cancer fighting phytonutrients so you should focus on those. You can add fruits to sweeten the juice but it should not make up the whole of the juice.

- **Drink the amount that you would eat.** If you are eating carrots, for example, it takes about 4-6 large carrots to make up to 8 ounces of carrot juice. This is a lot of carrots and more than you would likely eat if they were eaten whole. Only juice a couple of whole carrots at a time.

- **Add protein and fat to your diet.** Along with your juice (or in it), you should have some protein and healthy fats. This could mean that you eat yogurt with your juice or that you eat a handful of seeds or nuts. Eggs are also a good source of protein.

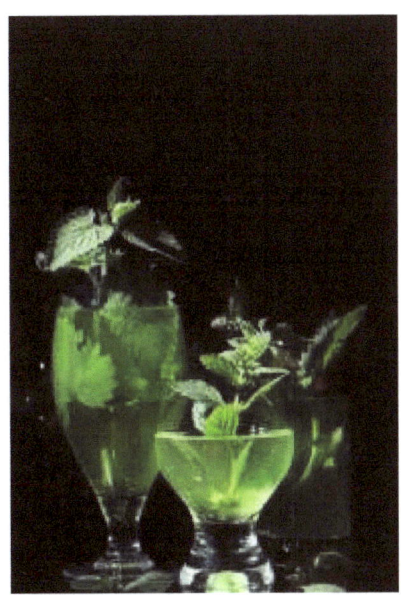

- **Don't forget the cruciferous vegetables**
  - Arugula
  - Broccoli
  - Bok Choy
  - Brussels Sprouts
  - Cabbage

- Kale
- Radishes
- Rutabaga
- Turnips
- Watercress
- Cauliflower
- Collard Greens

These can be juiced or eaten whole and contain many cancer fighting phytonutrients. Try eating at least 3 servings of cruciferous vegetables in your diet every day.

27 Healthy Juice Recipes

There are several juicing recipes made from a variety of fruits and vegetables. Here are 27 of my favorites:

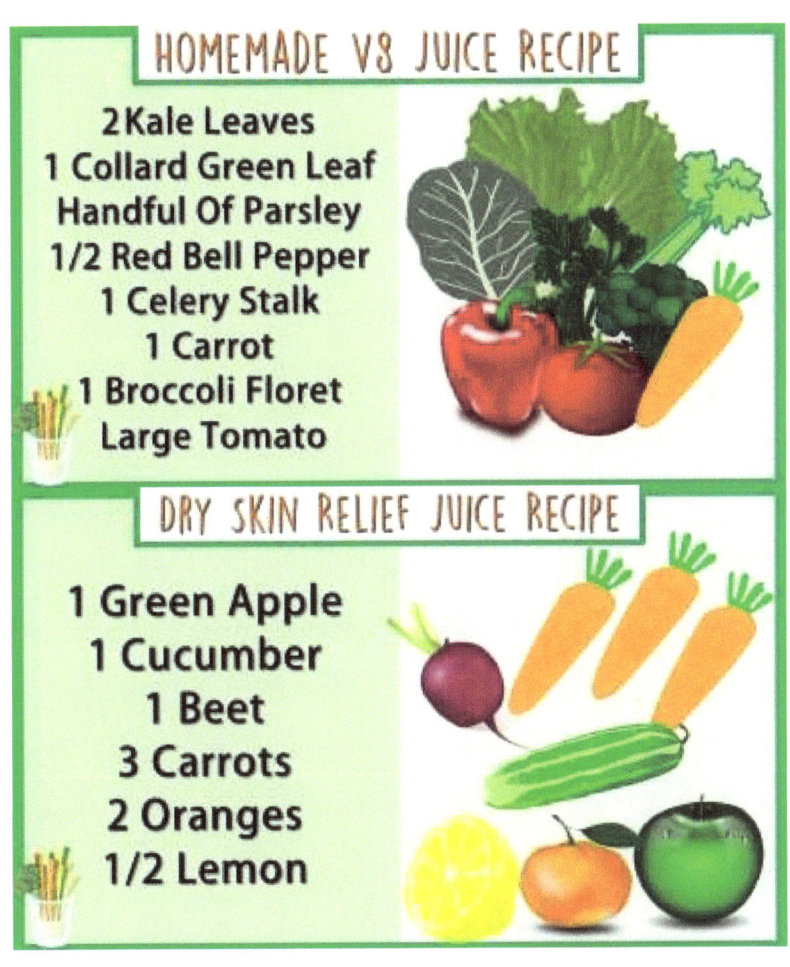

HOMEMADE V8 JUICE RECIPE

2 Kale Leaves
1 Collard Green Leaf
Handful Of Parsley
1/2 Red Bell Pepper
1 Celery Stalk
1 Carrot
1 Broccoli Floret
Large Tomato

DRY SKIN RELIEF JUICE RECIPE

1 Green Apple
1 Cucumber
1 Beet
3 Carrots
2 Oranges
1/2 Lemon

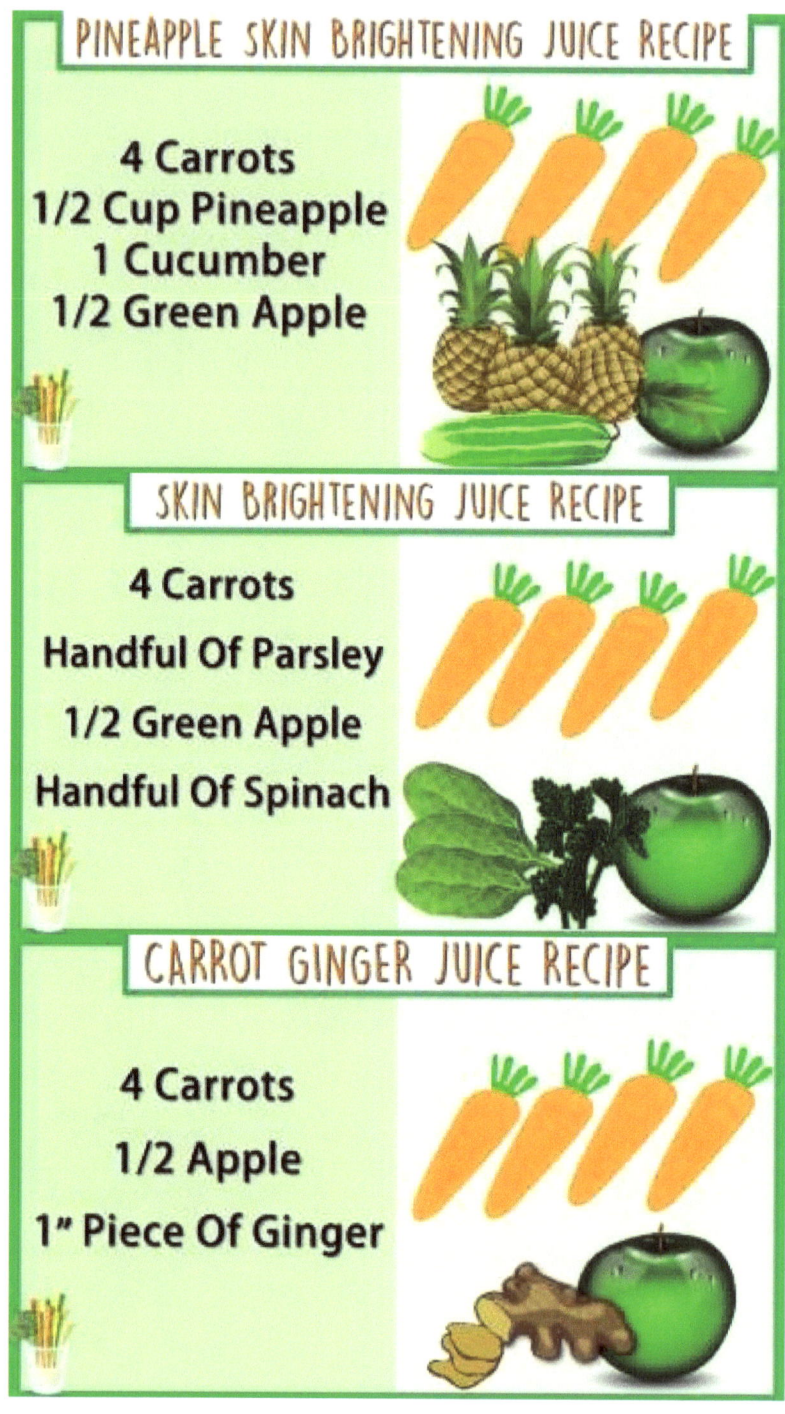

PINEAPPLE SKIN BRIGHTENING JUICE RECIPE

4 Carrots
1/2 Cup Pineapple
1 Cucumber
1/2 Green Apple

SKIN BRIGHTENING JUICE RECIPE

4 Carrots

Handful Of Parsley

1/2 Green Apple

Handful Of Spinach

CARROT GINGER JUICE RECIPE

4 Carrots

1/2 Apple

1" Piece Of Ginger

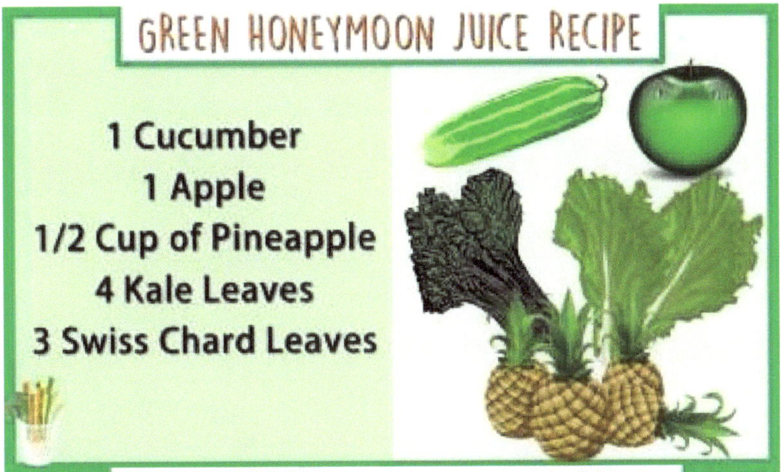

GREEN HONEYMOON JUICE RECIPE

1 Cucumber
1 Apple
1/2 Cup of Pineapple
4 Kale Leaves
3 Swiss Chard Leaves

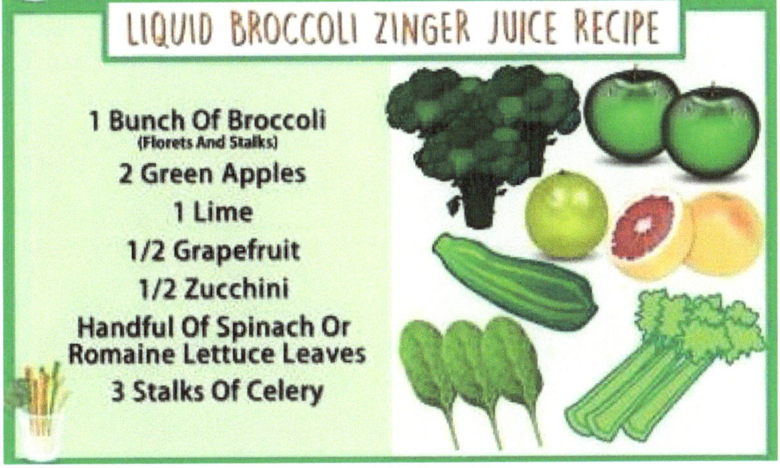

LIQUID BROCCOLI ZINGER JUICE RECIPE

1 Bunch Of Broccoli
(Florets And Stalks)
2 Green Apples
1 Lime
1/2 Grapefruit
1/2 Zucchini
Handful Of Spinach Or
Romaine Lettuce Leaves
3 Stalks Of Celery

GREEN JUICE CLEANSE RECIPE

4 Handfuls Of Spinach
3 Kale Leaves
2 Green Apples
3 Celery Stalks
1/2 Cucumber
1/2 Lemon

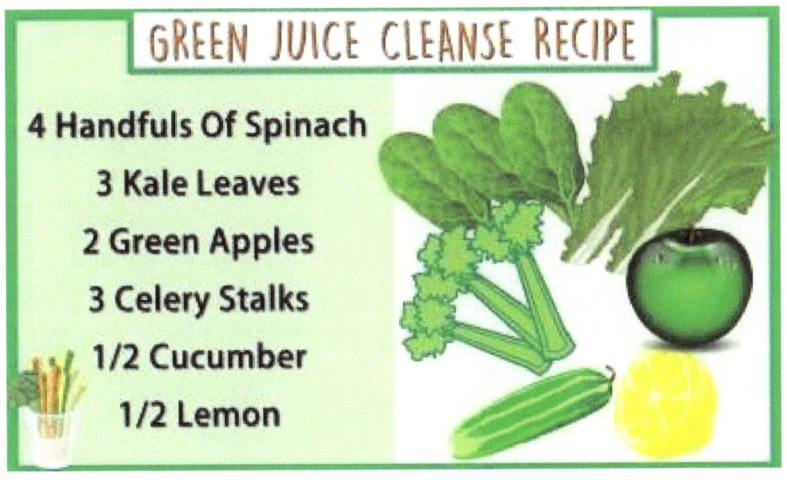

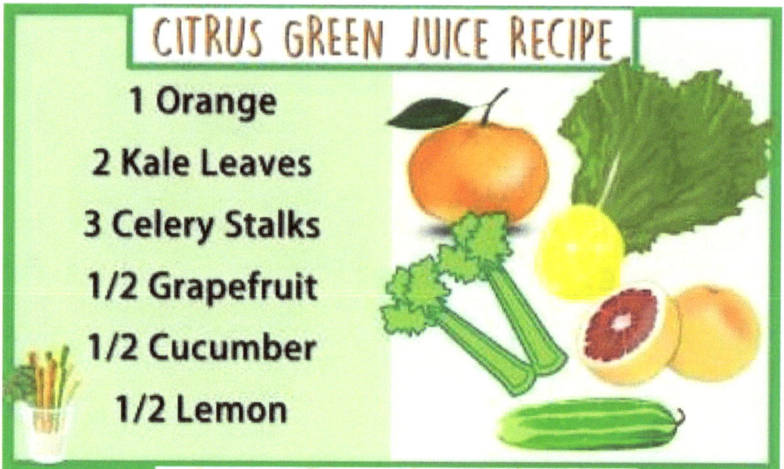

CITRUS GREEN JUICE RECIPE

1 Orange

2 Kale Leaves

3 Celery Stalks

1/2 Grapefruit

1/2 Cucumber

1/2 Lemon

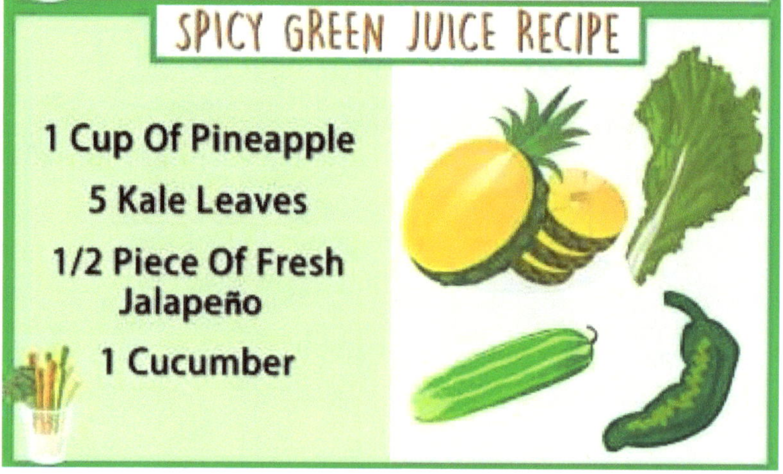

SPICY GREEN JUICE RECIPE

1 Cup Of Pineapple

5 Kale Leaves

1/2 Piece Of Fresh Jalapeño

1 Cucumber

MY SWEET BASIL JUICE RECIPE

1 Handful Of Basil

1 Apple

1 Cucumber

1/4 Lime

3 Spinach Leaves

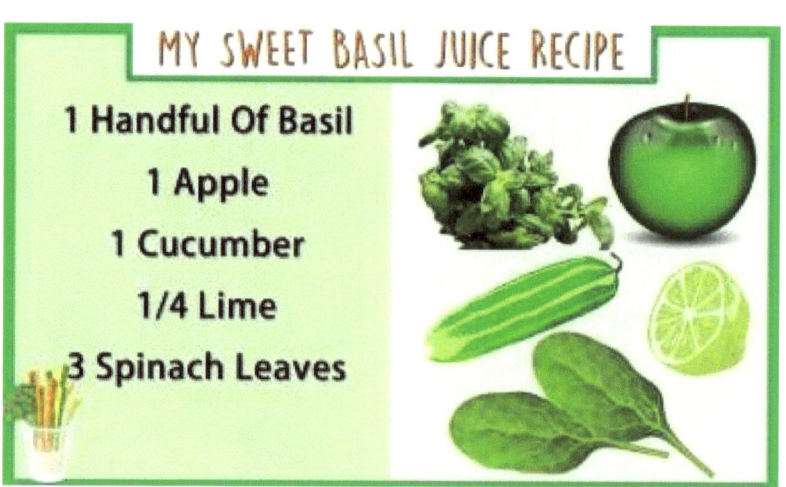

SWEET BERRY JUICE RECIPE

1. Juice 5 Kale Leaves
2. Blend 1 cup of strawberries and/or raspberries in a blender or food processor.
3. Add the berry puree to your kale juice, mix with a spoon and enjoy!

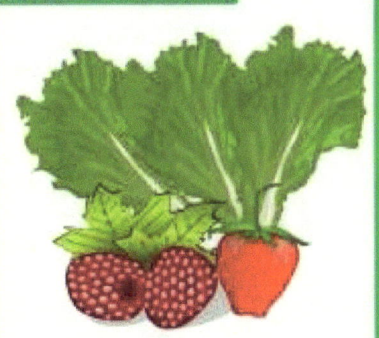

GREEN MORNING ENERGY JUICE RECIPE

5 Kale Leaves

1 Lemon

1 Apple

1" Piece Of Ginger

1 Sprig Of Mint

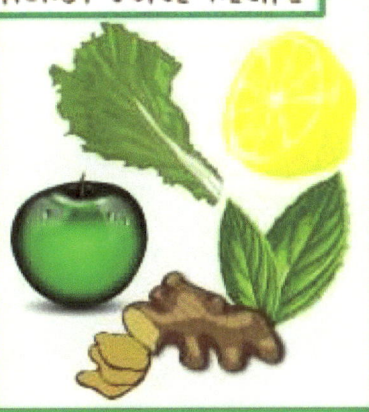

WATERMELON BREEZE JUICE RECIPE

2 Cups Of Watermelon

1 Cup Of Strawberries

1/2 Fresh Lime

1" Piece Of Ginger

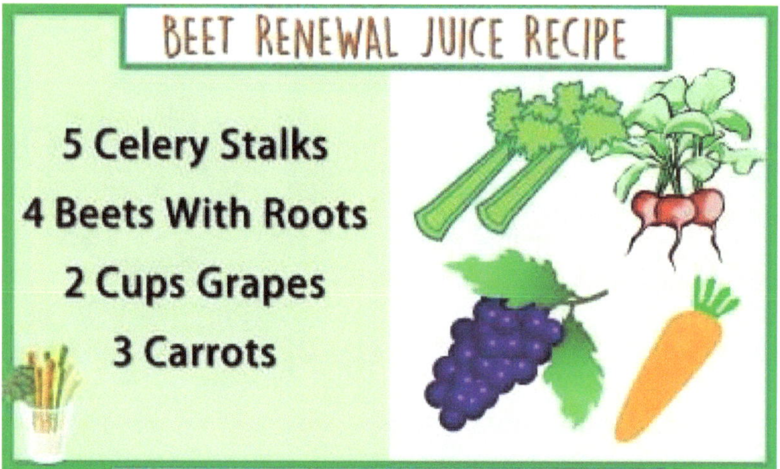

BEET RENEWAL JUICE RECIPE

5 Celery Stalks

4 Beets With Roots

2 Cups Grapes

3 Carrots

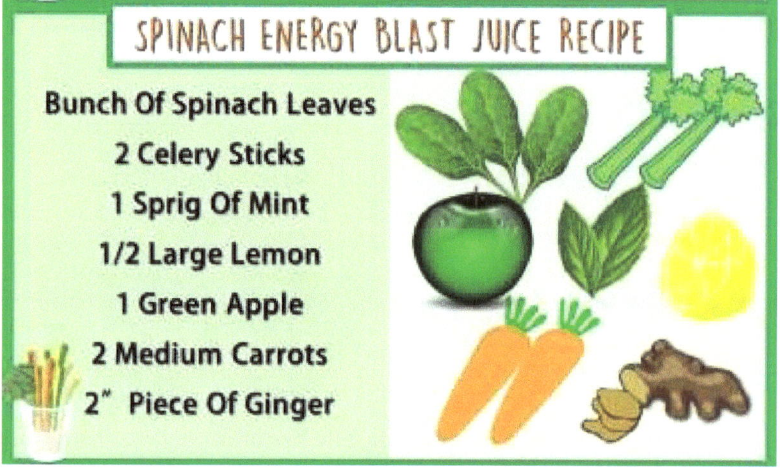

SPINACH ENERGY BLAST JUICE RECIPE

Bunch Of Spinach Leaves

2 Celery Sticks

1 Sprig Of Mint

1/2 Large Lemon

1 Green Apple

2 Medium Carrots

2" Piece Of Ginger

WHEATGRASS HARMONY JUICE RECIPE

3 Stalks Of Celery

2 Cucumbers

5 Spinach Leaves

1/2 Cup Fresh Parsley

2 Oz. Fresh
Wheatgrass Juice

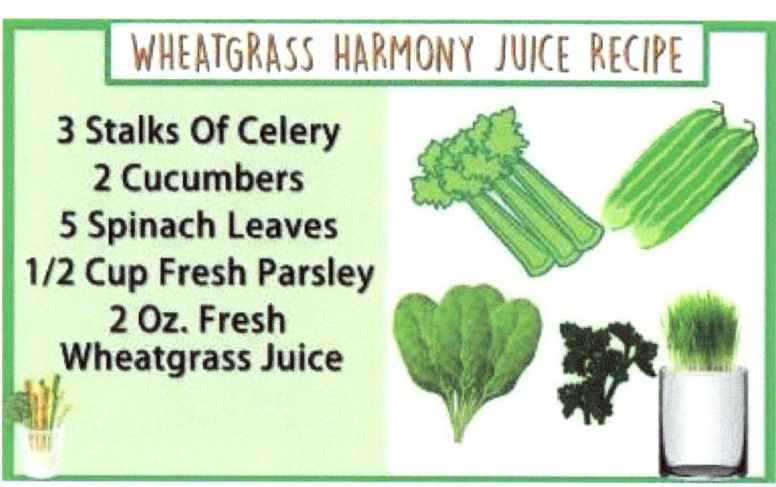

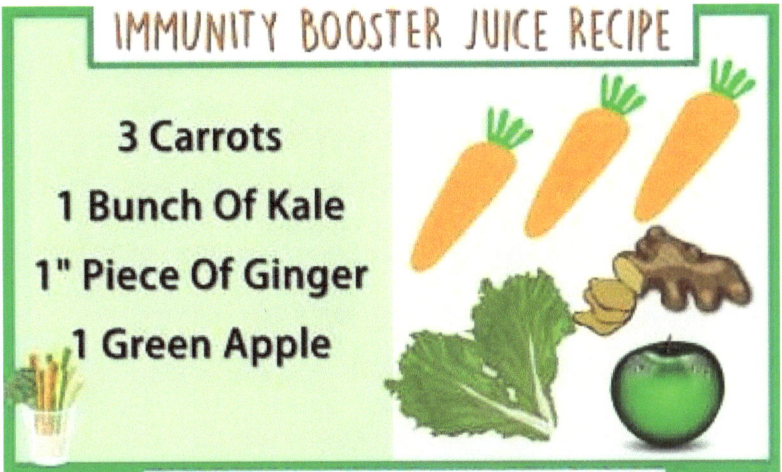

IMMUNITY BOOSTER JUICE RECIPE

3 Carrots
1 Bunch Of Kale
1" Piece Of Ginger
1 Green Apple

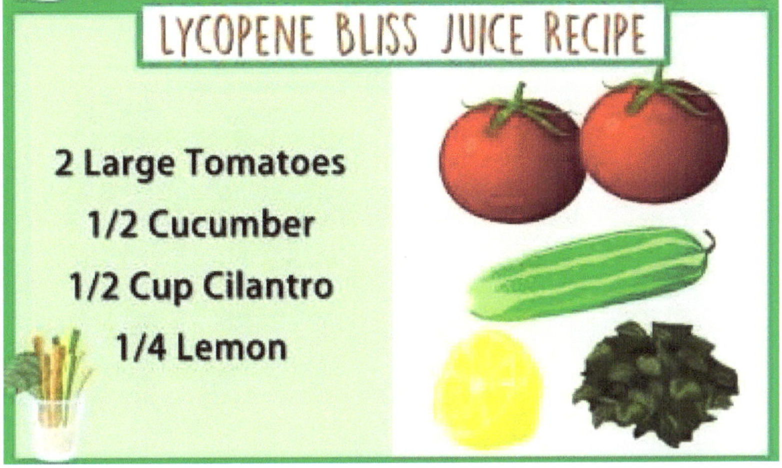

LYCOPENE BLISS JUICE RECIPE

2 Large Tomatoes
1/2 Cucumber
1/2 Cup Cilantro
1/4 Lemon

ENERGY BLAST JUICE RECIPE

3 Carrots
1 Green Apple
1 Peach
1/2 Lemon
1" Piece Of Ginger
1 Handful Of Mint Leaves

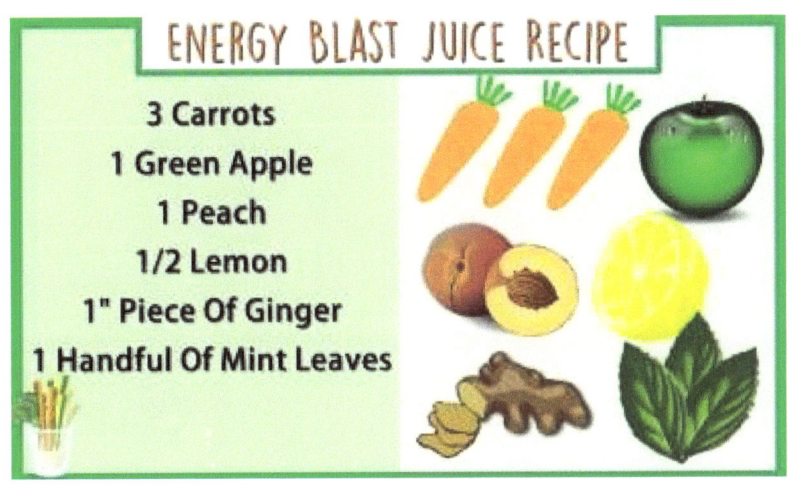

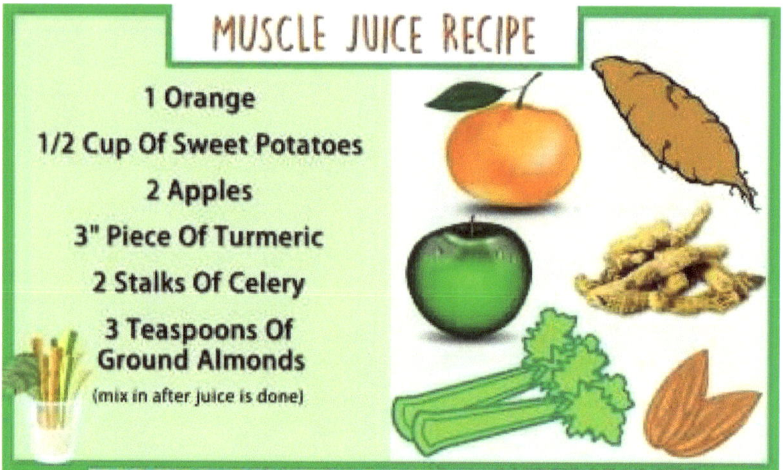

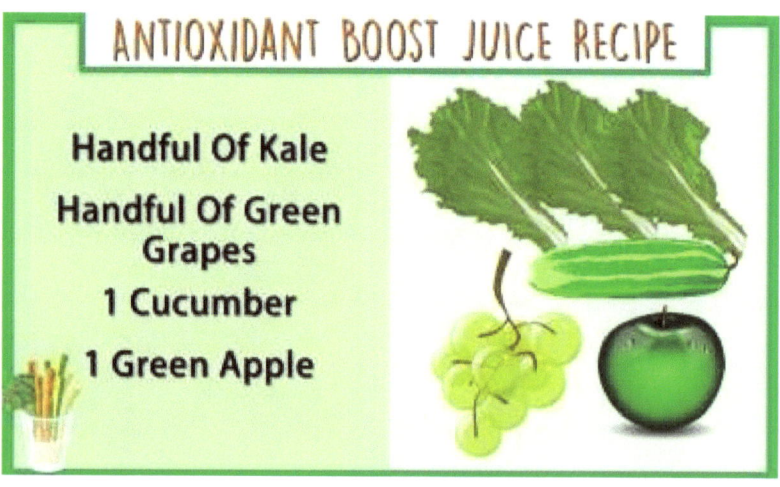

MUSCLE JUICE RECIPE

1 Orange
1/2 Cup Of Sweet Potatoes
2 Apples
3" Piece Of Turmeric
2 Stalks Of Celery
3 Teaspoons Of Ground Almonds
(mix in after juice is done)

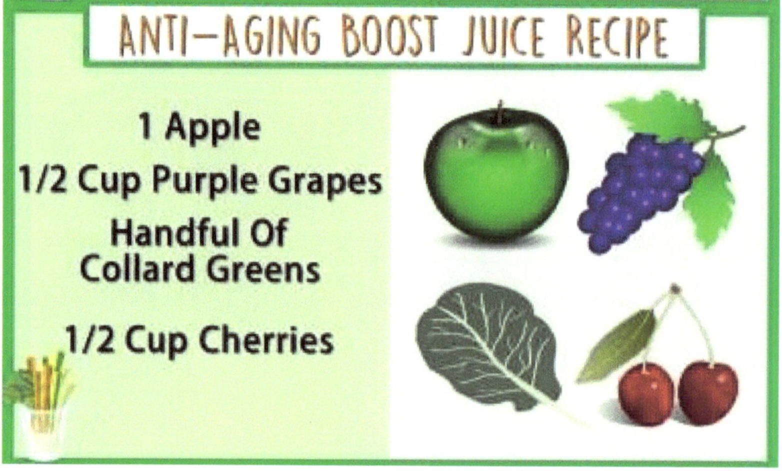

ANTI-AGING BOOST JUICE RECIPE

1 Apple
1/2 Cup Purple Grapes
Handful Of Collard Greens
1/2 Cup Cherries

ANTIOXIDANT BOOST JUICE RECIPE

Handful Of Kale
Handful Of Green Grapes
1 Cucumber
1 Green Apple

BEET TREAT JUICE RECIPE

1 Carrot
1 Beet
1" Pineapple Ring
1/2 Peeled Lemon
2 Green Apples
1" Piece Of Ginger

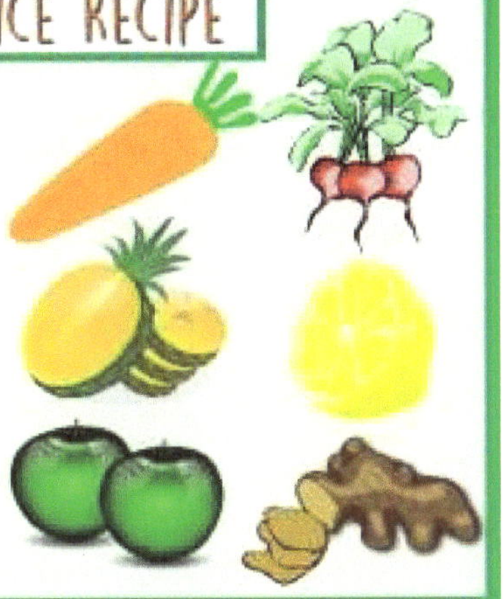

CARROT SPICE JUICE RECIPE

7 Carrots

1" Piece Of Ginger

1/2 Lime

1/4 Cup Cilantro

Pinch Of Cayenne Pepper
(Add To Finished Juice)

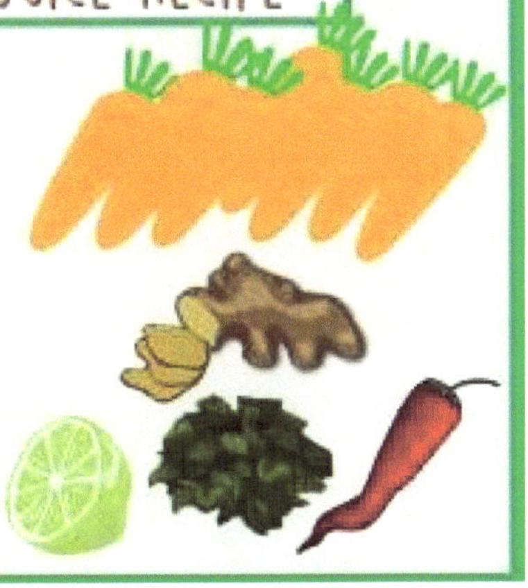

SWEET GREENS JUICE RECIPE

4 Kale Leaves

1 Green Apple

4 Celery Sticks

8 Parsley Sprigs

1 Cucumber

1/2 Lemon

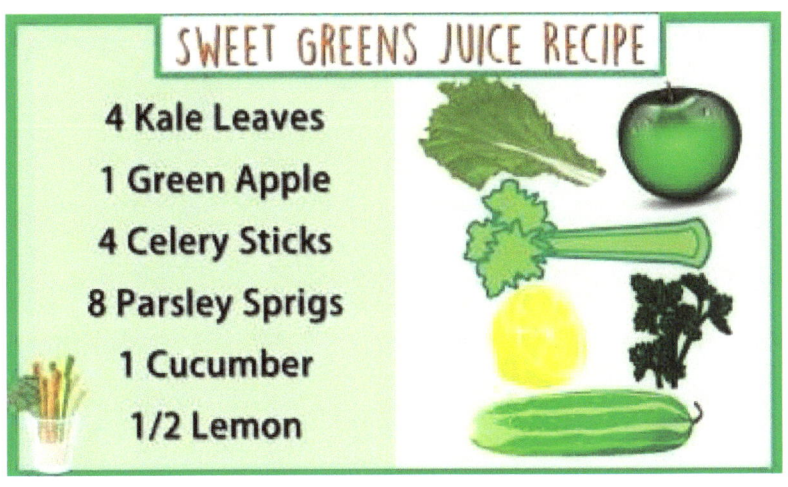

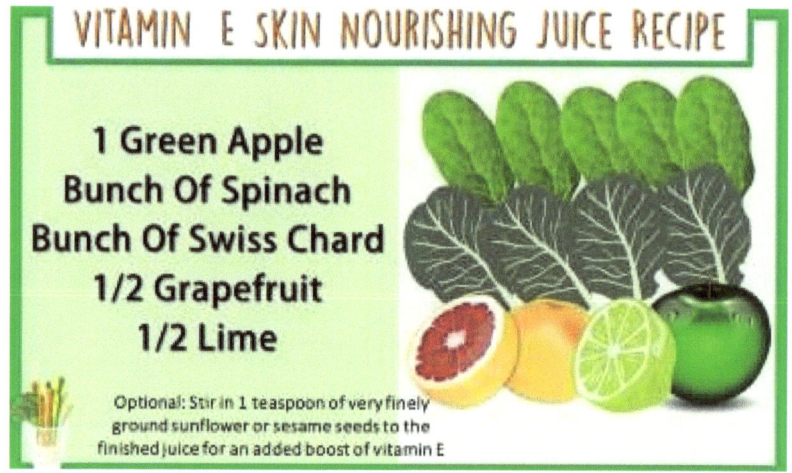

VITAMIN E SKIN NOURISHING JUICE RECIPE

1 Green Apple
Bunch Of Spinach
Bunch Of Swiss Chard
1/2 Grapefruit
1/2 Lime

Optional: Stir in 1 teaspoon of very finely
ground sunflower or sesame seeds to the
finished juice for an added boost of vitamin E

Other Senior Health and Fitness Books by This Author

If you would like to read more about Senior Health and Fitness, here is a list of the titles, CreateSpace links and descriptions:

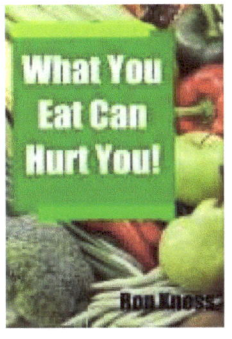

What You Eat Can Hurt You

https://www.createspace.com/4963196

Do you know that certain foods increase your risk for inflammation, disease and illness? It's true! And certain foods can help cure and heal you if you do get sick. Knowing which foods to eat and which ones to avoid empowers you to manage your own health.

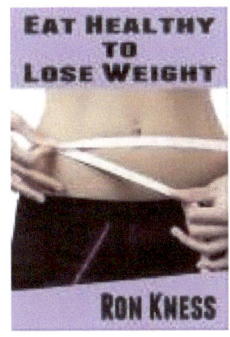

Eat Healthy to Lose Weight

https://www.createspace.com/4962939

As you read through our book, we show you which foods you should and should not be eating to reach your weight loss goal, along with discussing how to maintain your weight loss and stay within a few pounds of your goal weight. Banish the weight you keep gaining back each time by learning how to live a healthy lifestyle.

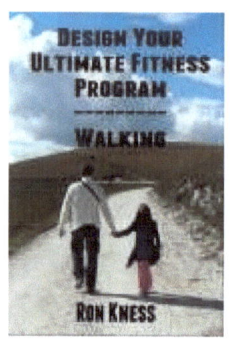

[Design Your Ultimate Fitness Program - Walking](https://www.createspace.com/5252272)

https://www.createspace.com/5252272

In my book Design Your Ultimate Fitness Program – Walking, we discuss the considerations that need to be made when designing a custom walking program, along with:

• Equipment needed
• Wearable technology you can use to track your walking
• And how to make walking more challenging

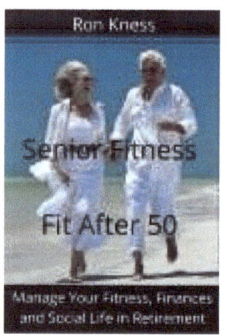

[Senior Fitness – Fit After 50: Learn How to Manage Your Fitness, Finances and Social Life in Retirement](https://www.createspace.com/5474751)

https://www.createspace.com/5474751

Inside you will discover answers to your most pressing questions:
• What do I need to know about downsizing my home?
• What are the best tips for staying healthy as you approach your 50's?
• When should I start planning for retirement?
• I am worried about being lonely once I retire, do others feel the same?
• Is it worthwhile to carry two homes during retirement?
And more…

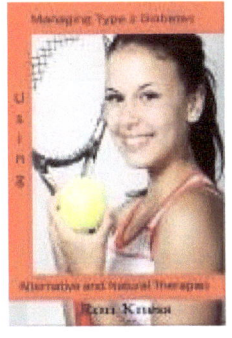

Managing Type 2 Diabetes Using Alternative And Natural Therapies

https://www.createspace.com/5401244

While Type 2 diabetes can be managed medically, there are many alternative natural and holistic methods of therapy and treatment that can further enhance quality of life and minimize the effects of this disease. In this book, I discuss 12 different types, including yoga, reflexology and acupuncture to name just three.

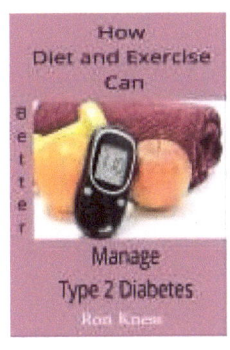

How Diet and Exercise Can Better Manage Type 2 Diabetes

https://www.createspace.com/5404845

Of the different types of diabetes, only Type 2 can be reversed. In my book How Diet and Exercise Can Better Manage Type 2 Diabetes, we reveal the three things you can do to best manage your disease, including:
• Diet
• Exercise
• Weight management

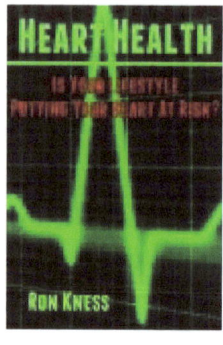

Heart Health: Is Your Lifestyle Putting Your Heart at Risk?

https://www.createspace.com/5464020

In my ebook Is Your Lifestyle Putting Your Heart At Risk? we discuss the six greatest risks to your heart and the lifestyle changes you can make to mitigate them.

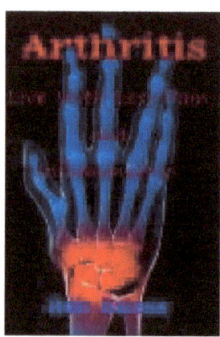

Arthritis – Live Wth Less Pain and Inflammation: Tips and Techniques You Can Use to Lessen the Pain and Inflammation

https://www.createspace.com/5457441

Discover Simple Tips & Information That Will Help Reduce The Painful Symptoms Of Arthritis!

You learn things like:
• Simple and effective information that will help you manage the pain and inflammation that comes along with arthritis, so that you can live an active, full life without debilitating pain.
• The different types of arthritis, their symptoms and how to alleviate their painful side effects.
• The pros and cons of over-the-counter arthritis medications, plus simple tips that will help you know how to choose the right supplements.
• Free, yet effective ways to get relief from arthritis pain and inflammation, so you don't have to suffer anymore.

the effects arthritis can have significant impact on your physical and mental well-being, but this books shows you how to overcome its painful symptoms and live life relatively pain free.

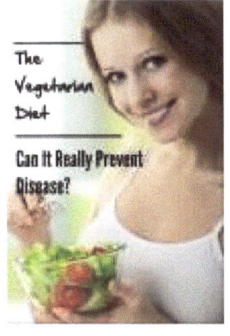

The Vegetarian Diet – Can It Really Prevent Disease?

https://www.createspace.com/5519874

Is a vegetarian diet right for you? Multiple studies have shown over and over that a vegetarian diet goes along way in preventing certain chronic diseases, such as:

• Heart Disease
• Cancer
• Diverticulitis
• Type 2 Diabetes
• Hypertension
• Obesity
• Kidney Failure

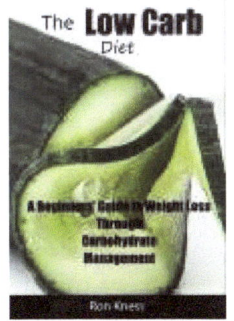

The Low Carb Diet: A Beginner's Guide to Weight Loss Through Carbohydrate Management

https://www.createspace.com/5416348

In my book "The Low-Carb Diet – A Beginners' Guide to Weight Loss Through Carbohydrate Management", I reveal a successful method of losing weight based in part on the amount and type of carbohydrates you consume.

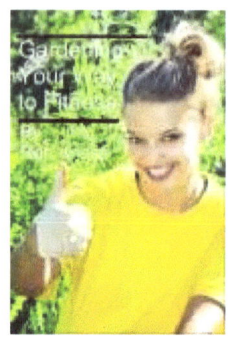

Gardening Your Way to Fitness: The Fun Way to Get Fit and Provide Beauty and Healthful Bounty for Your Family

https://www.createspace.com/5459564

The gym is a great place to stay fit during the colder seasons, but once the temperature turns warmer you want to spend more time outside. Plus, you'll have the benefit of fresh wholesome produce to enjoy by growing vegetables in your backyard garden.

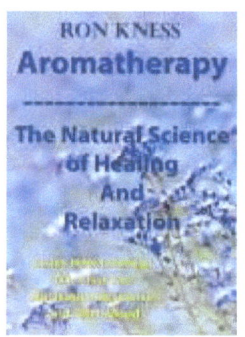

Aromatherapy - The Science of Healing and Relaxation: Learn How Essential Oils Elicit The Relaxation Response And Alter Mood

https://www.createspace.com/5714434

In my book Aromatherapy – The Science of Healing and Relaxation, we reveal the natural holistics methods you can use to heal the body from certain medical issues and to relive stress through relaxation. In particular we talk about:
• Aromatherapy - what it is and how it works
• Essential Oils – how the effects of certain aromas differs from others
• Recipes – how to make your own essential oil combinations

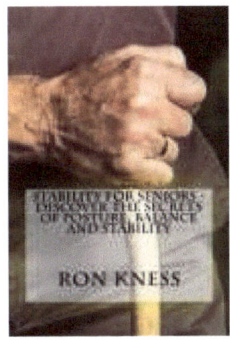

Stability for Seniors: Discover the Secrets of Posture, Balance and Stability

https://www.createspace.com/6096479

Many people sacrifice their health in pursuit of their career. They are so busy making a living that they neglect to make a life. The excuse that they do not have time to exercise is tossed about so frequently that they end up letting their health and fitness slide.

If you are not regularly active, you will have muscular atrophy over time. Your flexibility will decrease. Your core strength will diminish. As time progresses, you will be less limber and more rigid.

This is exactly how people age poorly. It's a process that has snowballed over time.

Only with regular exercise and a healthy diet can you have a body that is fit and has the ability to almost reverse aging.

If you have neglected your health for years and life seems to be a chore now because you can't get around without assistance, do not feel dejected.

You can remedy the situation. You can restore the strength, balance and stamina that you have lost. It is never too late to become what you might have been.

This guide will show you exactly what you need to do to restore your balance, strengthen your core and give you the ability to live life to its fullest. Read how …

About the Author

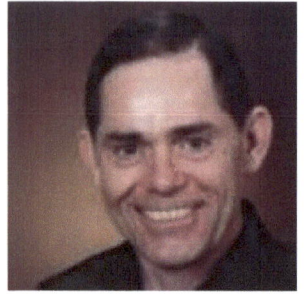

I grew up in Central Minnesota, where my parents own and operated a fishing resort. Once out of high school I tried a couple of semesters of college, only to quit halfway through the Spring term; I decided at that time that college wasn't for me.

Then I decided to follow my father's previous occupation as an auto mechanic. I graduated from a two-year of vocational training course and worked as a mechanic. While in vocational training, I decided to join the National Guard where I eventually ended up working full-time for 32 years.

So how does all of this relate to writing? In one of my leadership schools, the instructor, who was an English teacher at a juvenile detention center, presented writing to me in a whole new way - a way that started to develop my interest in working with words.

Fast forward about 40 years and I now have over 50 books listed on Amazon for Kindle and CreateSpace.

www.ingramcontent.com/pod-product-compliance
Lightning Source LLC
Chambersburg PA
CBHW050840290526
45792CB00001B/472